I0781516

"Enjoy and Lose Weight: Delicious Solutions"

Welcome to an exciting journey towards health and ideal weight! Transform your life by leaving stress and guilt over calories in the past!

Every meal counts! We will provide you with ideas for a balanced breakfast, lunch, and dinner. Learn how to plan a menu that meets your needs for proteins, carbohydrates, and fiber. **We will also discuss foods that can be eaten without the risk of weight gain and offer 43 recipes for healthy eating and weight loss. The book offers 10 healthy snacks and a sweet bonus - 30 recipes for delicious, sweet, but healthy desserts.**

In this book, we offer not just a weight loss plan but a comprehensive set of knowledge and practical recommendations for achieving long-term results. Approach the weight loss process with intelligence, not to suffer, and discover how healthy eating can change your life.

This book will be your reliable companion on the path to a healthy lifestyle. With its help, you will not only learn to eat right but also enjoy the process. Discover the secrets of effective weight loss and enjoy every moment of your journey to health!

Start your journey to a healthy body today with our practical plan and tasty recipes!

"The satisfaction of the most exotic dessert is nothing compared to the satisfaction of buying a smaller dress." —June Westyn

Table of contents

Chapter 1: Introduction to Healthy Eating and Weight Loss

Weight loss is not just a matter of appearance but also of healthy living. Many people strive to lose weight to feel better, live longer, and avoid obesity-related diseases. However, the path to a healthy body does not lie through fasting or extreme diets but through understanding and applying the principles of proper and balanced nutrition.

Why Diets Don't Work?

Most diets focus on short-term results, offering rapid weight loss through dietary restrictions. However, such approaches often lead to the opposite effect—weight returns and sometimes even increases. This happens because the body starts to store fats when it experiences a calorie deficit. Additionally, strict restrictions lead to a lack of essential vitamins and minerals, which can harm health.

Basics of Healthy Eating

Healthy eating is not a diet but a lifestyle. It is based on a balanced intake of proteins, fats, and carbohydrates, as well as the right choice and quantity of foods. This approach provides the body with everything it needs for normal functioning, helps maintain a healthy weight, and improves overall well-being.

Here are some interesting facts about healthy eating:

1. **Nuts and Seeds Are Superfoods**: Although they are often considered calorie-dense, research shows that nuts and seeds can aid in weight loss. They are rich in healthy fats, protein, and fiber, making them a great snack that keeps hunger at bay for longer.

2. **Color of Vegetables Matters**: Different colors of fruits and vegetables reflect different types of antioxidants and nutrients. For example, bright red tomatoes are rich in lycopene, which is beneficial for heart health, while orange carrots contain beta-carotene, which is good for vision.

3. **Water Helps Burn Calories**: Drinking water before meals can help you eat less and speed up your metabolism. Studies show that drinking 500 ml of water can increase metabolism by 24-30% for 1.5 hours.

4. **Dark Chocolate Is a Great Source of Antioxidants**: Dark chocolate with high cocoa content not only satisfies sweet cravings but is also rich in antioxidants that can help improve heart health and boost mood.

5. **Yogurt Is Good for Digestion**: Probiotics found in yogurt and other fermented products promote the growth of beneficial bacteria in the gut, which aids digestion and supports immune system health.

6. **Olive Oil Is the "Liquid Gold" of the Mediterranean**: Extra virgin olive oil is a cornerstone of the Mediterranean diet, one of the healthiest in the world. It is rich in monounsaturated fats and antioxidants, which reduce the risk of cardiovascular diseases.

7. **Green Tea Is a Longevity Drink**: Green tea is rich in antioxidants known as catechins, which help protect cells from damage and may reduce the risk of chronic diseases.

8. **Leafy Greens Are Key to Longevity**: Leafy green vegetables like spinach and kale are packed with vitamins, minerals, and antioxidants. Regular consumption is linked to improved heart and brain health.

9. **Diet Affects Mood**: Certain foods, such as fatty fish (rich in omega-3), nuts, berries, and whole grains, can improve mood and help combat depression.

10. **Chewing Food Slowly Helps You Eat Less**: The brain takes about 20 minutes to recognize that the stomach is full. Chewing food slowly helps you understand when you are full before overeating.

Chapter 2: What Are Macronutrients and Micronutrients?

1. What Are Macronutrients and Micronutrients?

- **Macronutrients** are the nutrients that the body requires in large amounts: proteins, fats, and carbohydrates. They provide the energy necessary for maintaining vital functions.

- **Micronutrients** are vitamins and minerals needed in smaller quantities but play a crucial role in maintaining health.

Key Macronutrients

1. **Proteins**

   - **Functions**: Tissue building, cell repair, involvement in immune processes.

   - **Sources**: Meat, fish, eggs, legumes, nuts.

   - **Impact on Weight Loss**: Increasing protein intake helps maintain muscle mass and promotes fat burning.

2. **Fats**

   - **Functions**: Energy provision, vitamin absorption, organ protection.

   - **Sources**: Olive oil, nuts, avocado, fatty fish.

   - **Impact on Weight Loss**: Healthy fats contribute to a feeling of fullness and support hormonal balance.

3. **Carbohydrates**

   - **Functions**: The primary source of energy for the brain and muscles.

   - **Sources**: Whole grains, vegetables, fruits.

   - **Impact on Weight Loss**: Slow carbohydrates with a low glycemic index help control appetite and blood sugar levels.

Key Micronutrients

1. **Vitamins**

   - **Vitamin D**: Strengthens bones, supports the immune system.
     - **Sources**: Fish oil, mushrooms, sunlight.
   - **Vitamin B12**: Involved in the formation of red blood cells and the nervous system.
     - **Sources**: Meat, fish, dairy products.
   - **Vitamin C**: Antioxidant, promotes wound healing, strengthens immunity.
     - **Sources**: Citrus fruits, berries, broccoli.

2. **Minerals**

   - **Calcium**: Necessary for strong bones and teeth, involved in muscle contractions.
     - **Sources**: Dairy products, greens, almonds.
   - **Iron**: Important for oxygen transport in the blood.
     - **Sources**: Red meat, spinach, legumes.
   - **Magnesium**: Regulates muscle and nerve functions, helps control blood sugar levels.
     - **Sources**: Nuts, seeds, dark chocolate.

The Role of Balance

- Including all necessary macro- and micronutrients in the right proportions in your diet helps not only maintain health but also effectively lose weight by improving metabolism and reducing the risk of deficiencies.

Facts About Macronutrients

1. **Proteins and Calorie Burning**: Digesting protein requires more energy than processing fats and carbohydrates. This means that the body burns more calories digesting protein-rich foods, which can aid in weight loss.

2. **Fats and the Brain**: The human brain is 60% fat, and omega-3 fatty acids are particularly important for its normal functioning. They improve memory and cognitive functions.

3. **Carbohydrates and Mood**: Carbohydrates promote the production of serotonin, a neurotransmitter that improves mood and helps fight depression. Therefore, completely cutting out carbohydrates can negatively affect emotional well-being.

Facts About Micronutrients

1. **Vitamin D and Sunlight**: Our body can produce vitamin D on its own, but only under the influence of sunlight. During the winter months, many people experience a deficiency of this vitamin, which can weaken the immune system and cause fatigue.

2. **Iron and Energy**: Iron deficiency is one of the most common causes of chronic fatigue. Iron is necessary for the formation of hemoglobin, which carries oxygen to the cells. Without enough oxygen, the body starts to work less efficiently.

3. **Magnesium and Stress**: Magnesium is known as the "anti-stress" mineral because it helps relax muscles and reduce cortisol levels—the stress hormone. A lack of magnesium can increase anxiety and tension.

4. **Calcium and Muscle Cramps**: A lack of calcium can lead to muscle cramps and spasms, as calcium is involved in the processes of muscle contraction and relaxation.

5. **Vitamin C and Collagen**: Vitamin C plays a key role in the synthesis of collagen, which supports the health of the skin, joints, and blood vessels.

Without enough vitamin C, the skin loses its elasticity and becomes more prone to damage.

Additional Interesting Facts

1. **Bioavailability of Micronutrients**: Some micronutrients are better absorbed in the presence of others. For example, vitamin C significantly increases the absorption of iron from plant-based foods.

2. **Salt and Iodine**: Iodine deficiency was once widespread in many countries, leading to thyroid diseases. Today, iodized salt helps prevent this deficiency.

Chapter 3: Is Portion Control and Calorie Counting Necessary?

Portion Sizes Portion control is one of the key aspects of the weight loss process. Often, we overeat without realizing how many calories we are consuming. Using small plates, measuring portions, and eating slowly can help avoid overeating.

Calorie Counting Calorie counting is one of the most effective methods of weight control, but it is not the only way to lose weight. Let's consider both approaches:

Why Calorie Counting Can Help:

1. **Control Over Intake:** Calorie counting helps you be aware of how much energy you consume from food and compare it with how much energy you expend. This allows you to regulate portions and avoid overeating.

2. **Creating a Calorie Deficit:** To lose weight, you need to create a calorie deficit, which means consuming less energy than your body uses. Calorie counting helps you understand exactly how deficit your diet is.

3. **Food Choices:** Calorie counting encourages choosing lower-calorie and nutritious foods, such as vegetables, fruits, lean proteins, and whole grains.

Why You Can Manage Without Calorie Counting:

1. **Mindful Eating:** The practice of mindful eating involves paying attention to hunger and fullness signals, choosing nutritious foods, and avoiding emotional eating. This approach helps control weight without strict calorie counting.

2. **Choosing Healthy Foods:** If you choose nutritious and low-calorie foods (e.g., vegetables, lean meats, fish), you can eat to satiety without worrying about gaining weight. Such foods are rich in fiber, protein, and water, making them filling and low in calories.

3. **Reasonable Portion Control:** Portion control can be a simple and intuitive way to maintain a calorie deficit without having to count every calorie. Using

smaller plates, avoiding second helpings, and steering clear of snacking between meals can be effective enough.

Calorie counting is a useful tool for those who want to have precise control over their diet. However, for many people, following general principles of healthy eating, mindful food consumption, and reasonable portion control can be effective enough for achieving and maintaining a healthy weight. The main thing is to find an approach that is sustainable and comfortable for you in the long term.

What Should Be the Weight of a Single Portion Per Meal?

The portion size for one meal can vary depending on individual calorie needs, physical activity level, and weight loss goals. However, there are general recommendations to help determine what the weight of one portion should be:

General Recommendations for Portion Sizes:

1. **Vegetables:**
   - Recommended portion weight: 150-200 g.
   - Vegetables should make up a significant part of your plate. They are low in calories, rich in fiber, vitamins, and minerals.

2. **Protein Foods:**
   - Recommended portion weight: 100-150 g of the cooked product (e.g., meat, fish, eggs, cottage cheese).
   - Protein helps maintain muscle mass and a feeling of fullness.

3. **Grains and Carbohydrates:**
   - Recommended portion weight: 50-100 g (e.g., cooked grains, bread, potatoes).
   - Carbohydrates should make up about a quarter of your plate. Choose whole grains that contain more fiber.

4. **Fruits:**

- o   Recommended portion weight: 100-150 g.

- o   Fruits can be a healthy part of the diet, especially if used as a snack or added to main dishes.

5. **Fats:**

- o   Recommended portion weight: 10-20 g (e.g., oils, nuts, avocado).

- o   Fats are necessary for the normal functioning of the body, but their amount should be limited due to their high caloric content.

How to Determine Portion Size Without a Scale:

- **Palm Size:** A portion of protein (meat, fish) is roughly equivalent to the size and thickness of your palm.

- **Fist Size:** A portion of vegetables or fruits can be about the size of your fist.

- **Handful:** A portion of carbohydrates (grains, pasta) should fit in one handful

- **Thumb:** A portion of fats, such as oils or nuts, should be about the size of your thumb.

Portion size depends on your overall calorie intake and goals, but following these recommendations will help you balance your diet and maintain a healthy weight. It is important to remember that you should feel full but not overwhelmed after eating, and avoid excessively large portions that can lead to overeating.

How to Learn to Count Calories

Learning to count calories is an important step for those who want to control their weight and diet. Here's a simple and understandable way to master this skill:

1. **Determine Your Daily Calorie Requirement:**

- o   **Basal Metabolic Rate (BMR):** This is the number of calories your body needs at rest. The Harris-Benedict formula can help you calculate BMR:

- For men:

    - **Metric (kg and cm):** BMR = 88.36 + (13.4 × weight in kg) + (4.8 × height in cm) - (5.7 × age in years)

    - **Imperial (lbs and inches):** BMR = 66 + (6.23 × weight in lbs) + (12.7 × height in inches) - (6.8 × age in years)

- For women:

    - **Metric (kg and cm):** BMR = 447.6 + (9.2 × weight in kg) + (3.1 × height in cm) - (4.3 × age in years)

    - **Imperial (lbs and inches):** BMR = 655 + (4.35 × weight in lbs) + (4.7 × height in inches) - (4.7 × age in years)

- **Total Daily Energy Expenditure (TDEE):** TDEE = BMR × Physical Activity Level:

    - **Physical Activity Levels:**

    - Sedentary (little or no exercise): TDEE = BMR × 1.2

    - Lightly active (light exercise 1-3 times/week): TDEE = BMR × 1.375

    - Moderately active (moderate exercise 3-5 times/week): TDEE = BMR × 1.55

    - Very active (hard exercise 6-7 times/week): TDEE = BMR × 1.725

    - Extremely active (very hard exercise or physical job): TDEE = BMR × 1.9

Example Calculation: Suppose you are a woman, weighing 150 lbs, 65 inches tall, 30 years old, and moderately active:

- BMR using the imperial formula: BMR = 655 + (4.35 × 150) + (4.7 × 65) - (4.7 × 30) = 655 + 652.5 + 305.5 - 141 = 1472 kcal

- TDEE for moderate activity: TDEE = 1472 × 1.55 = 2271 kcal

If using metric units:

- o BMR using the metric formula: BMR = 447.6 + (9.2 × 68) + (3.1 × 165) - (4.3 × 30) = 447.6 + 625.6 + 511.5 - 129 = 1455.7 kcal

- o TDEE for moderate activity: TDEE = 1455.7 × 1.55 = 2256.3 kcal

Both formulas will give you similar results, and you can choose the one that is more convenient for you to use.

2. **Use a Nutrition App or Food Diary:**

   - o Apps can help you track calories. You simply enter the foods you eat, and the app calculates their caloric content.

   - o If you prefer manual counting, keep a diary and write down the number of calories for each meal.

3. **Learn to Read Labels:**

   - o Food packaging indicates the number of calories per 100 grams or per serving. It's important to understand that often the package contains multiple servings.

   - o Pay attention to serving sizes and compare them to what you actually eat.

4. **Use Kitchen Scales:**

   - o For accurate calorie counting, it's important to know the exact weight of the food you eat. Kitchen scales will help you measure the portion and find out how many calories are in that amount of food.

5. **Memorize the Caloric Content of Basic Foods:**

   - o Gradually, you'll start remembering the caloric content of the foods you consume regularly. This will make counting easier and allow you to more accurately control your diet.

6. **Learn to Account for Complex Dishes:**

- o If a dish consists of multiple ingredients, calculate the caloric content of each one and add them up. For example, if you're making a salad, consider the calories of the vegetables, dressing, and any add-ins.

7. **Monitor Progress:**

- o It's important not only to count calories but also to track results. Regularly check your weight and adjust your diet as necessary.

At first, calorie counting may seem complicated, but with practice, it will become a habit. It's an excellent tool for understanding how much energy you are consuming and how it affects your weight.

Caloric Content of Some Basic Foods per 100 Grams

These data will help you better navigate calorie counting:

Protein Foods:

- Chicken breast (skinless): 110-120 kcal
- Beef (lean): 250-280 kcal
- Pork (lean): 230-260 kcal
- Cod (fish): 70-80 kcal
- Salmon: 200-220 kcal
- Cottage cheese (low-fat): 70-90 kcal
- Cottage cheese (full-fat): 150-170 kcal
- Egg (boiled): 140-150 kcal

Carbohydrate Foods:

- Rice (boiled, white): 110-130 kcal
- Buckwheat (boiled): 110-120 kcal
- Oatmeal (on water): 70-80 kcal
- Pasta (boiled): 110-130 kcal

- Potato (boiled): 75-85 kcal

- Bread (wheat): 240-270 kcal

- Bread (rye): 190-210 kcal

Fruits:

- Apple: 45-50 kcal

- Banana: 85-95 kcal

- Orange: 35-45 kcal

- Pear: 40-50 kcal

- Kiwi: 50-60 kcal

- Grapes: 65-75 kcal

Vegetables:

- Cucumbers: 10-15 kcal

- Tomatoes: 15-20 kcal

- Cabbage (white): 25-30 kcal

- Carrots: 30-40 kcal

- Beets: 40-45 kcal

- Broccoli: 30-35 kcal

Dairy Products:

- Milk (2.5%): 50-55 kcal

- Yogurt (plain, unsweetened): 60-70 kcal

- Kefir (1%): 35-40 kcal

- Cheese (hard, 45%): 350-400 kcal

Nuts and Seeds:

- Almonds: 570-600 kcal

- Walnuts: 650-670 kcal

- Sunflower seeds: 580-600 kcal

- Hazelnuts: 630-650 kcal

Drinks:

- Tea (without sugar): 1-2 kcal

- Coffee (black, without sugar): 2-5 kcal

- Orange juice (without sugar): 45-50 kcal

These figures are averages and may vary slightly depending on the specific product or method of preparation.

Meal Regularity

Regular meals help maintain blood sugar levels and prevent overeating. It is recommended to eat 3-4 times a day with intervals of 3-4 hours. This helps control appetite and maintain energy levels.

Hydration

Water plays an important role in the weight loss process. It helps speed up metabolism, remove toxins, and control appetite. It is recommended to drink at least 1.5-2 liters of water per day.

Chapter 4: How to Plan a Menu

Breakfast

Breakfast is the main meal that sets the tone for the entire day. It should be rich in proteins and complex carbohydrates. An example of a healthy breakfast: oatmeal with nuts and berries, or an omelet with vegetables.

Lunch

Lunch should include a variety of protein and fiber sources. A great option is baked chicken breast with quinoa and a fresh vegetable salad.

Dinner

Dinner should be light yet nutritious. It's best to choose foods that are easy to digest, such as fish with steamed vegetables.

Foods You Can Eat Without the Risk of Gaining Weight:

1. **Vegetables:**

   - **Broccoli, cauliflower, spinach, lettuce, cucumbers, celery:** These foods are high in fiber and water, which help create a feeling of fullness with a minimal number of calories.

   - **Zucchini, tomatoes, bell peppers:** Light and low-calorie vegetables that can be consumed in large quantities.

2. **Fruits:**

   - **Apples, grapefruits, berries (blueberries, raspberries, strawberries):** They contain a lot of fiber, which helps control appetite, and have a low glycemic index.

   - **Watermelon, melon:** These fruits are mostly water and have low calories, making them ideal for snacking.

3. **Protein Foods:**

- o **Chicken breast, turkey, eggs:** Protein sources that help maintain a feeling of fullness for longer.

    - o **Fish (especially white fish), seafood:** Low-calorie protein sources that are high in omega-3 fatty acids.

4. **Dairy Products:**

    - o **Low-fat cottage cheese, natural yogurt, kefir:** These products contain protein and beneficial probiotics that support digestion.

5. **Grains and Legumes:**

    - o **Oatmeal, quinoa, lentils, chickpeas:** These foods provide a long-lasting feeling of fullness due to their high fiber and protein content.

6. **Nuts and Seeds (in moderation):**

    - o **Almonds, walnuts, chia seeds, flax seeds:** They are rich in healthy fats, protein, and fiber, but due to their high calorie content, they should be consumed in small amounts.

7. **Liquids:**

    - o **Water, green tea, herbal teas, unsweetened compotes:** Calorie-free liquids help control hunger and maintain water balance.

These foods help control weight as they are low in calories but packed with essential nutrients. Including them in your diet can help avoid hunger and maintain energy throughout the day.

To avoid gaining weight, it is recommended to eliminate or significantly reduce the consumption of the following products:

1. Sugar and sweets:

• Sugar, candy, baked goods, fizzy drinks and sweet juices contain a lot of calories and few nutrients, which contributes to weight gain.

2. Processed foods:

• Semi-finished products, sausages, hot dogs, chips and ready meals usually contain a lot of hidden fats, sugar and salt, which also contributes to overeating.

3. White bread and baked goods made from refined flour:

• Products made from white flour have a high glycemic index, which leads to a sharp increase in blood sugar levels and a quick feeling of hunger.

4. Fatty dairy products:

• Full-fat milk, cream, fatty cheeses and yogurts can contain a lot of saturated fat, which increases the calorie content of the diet.

5. Fried foods:

• Foods cooked in deep fat or with a lot of oil are very caloric and can contribute to weight gain.

6 Alcohol:

• Alcoholic drinks are high in calories and can slow down your metabolism, making it harder to lose weight.

7 Fast Food:

• Most fast food is high in calories, fat, and sugar, but low in nutrients.

8 Sugary Breakfasts:

• Sugary cereals, granola bars with added sugar, and other processed grains often contain hidden sugars and are low in fiber.

Eliminating or limiting these foods from your diet and replacing them with healthier alternatives like fresh vegetables, fruits, whole grains, and lean proteins can help you manage your weight and improve your overall health.

Here are some healthy alternatives to foods that you should eliminate or reduce in your diet to control your weight:

1. Sugar and sweets:

• Alternative: Fruits (fresh or dried without sugar), berries, honey (in moderation), natural sweeteners (stevia, erythritol), dark chocolate (with high cocoa content).

2. Processed foods:

• Alternative: Homemade dishes made from fresh ingredients, natural meat and fish products (baked or steamed), nuts, seeds and natural yogurts without additives.

3. White bread and pastries made from refined flour:

• Alternative: Whole grain bread, rye bread, whole grain crispbread, oatmeal, brown rice, quinoa, bulgur, oat flakes.

4 Full-fat dairy products:

• Alternative: Skim or low-fat milk, low-fat Greek yogurt, low-fat cottage cheese, low-fat cheeses, plant-based milk alternatives (almond, coconut, soy milk without sugar).

5 Fried foods:

• Alternative: Baked, steamed or grilled dishes, stewed vegetables, baked potatoes in the oven with a minimum amount of oil, vegetable chips cooked in the oven.

6 Alcohol:

• Alternative: Water with lemon or lime, herbal teas, natural fruit and vegetable smoothies, non-alcoholic cocktails based on mineral water, kefir or yogurt.

7 Fast Food:

• Alternative: Homemade burgers made from lean meat or fish, salads with light dressings, vegetable dishes prepared at home, baked potato wedges made from sweet potatoes.

8 Sweet Breakfasts:

• <u>Alternative:</u> Oatmeal with fruits and nuts, whole grain cereal without sugar, Greek yogurt with berries and honey, omelet with vegetables, smoothies with added greens, avocado on whole grain toast.

Chapter 5: Recipes for 30 Dishes for Healthy Eating and Weight Loss

Meal Plan 1

Breakfast: Vegetable Omelette with Avocado

Ingredients:

- Eggs: 2 (120g / 4.2 oz)
- Milk: 50 ml / 1.7 oz
- Tomatoes: 1 (100g / 3.5 oz)
- Spinach: 50g / 1.7 oz
- Avocado: ½ (70g / 2.5 oz)
- Olive oil: 1 tsp (5 ml / 0.17 oz)
- Salt and pepper to taste

Instructions:

1. Whisk the eggs with milk in a bowl.
2. Heat olive oil in a pan.
3. Add chopped tomatoes and spinach, sauté for 2-3 minutes.
4. Pour the egg mixture into the pan and cook on medium heat until done, about 5-7 minutes.
5. Slice the avocado and serve it alongside the omelette.

Nutritional Information:

- Calories: 300 kcal
- Protein: 16g
- Fat: 24g
- Yield: 340g / 12 oz
- Cooking Time: 15 minutes
- Cooking Temperature: Medium heat

Lunch: Chicken Breast with Quinoa and Broccoli

Ingredients:

- Chicken breast: 200g / 7 oz
- Quinoa: 50g / 1.7 oz
- Broccoli: 150g / 5.3 oz
- Olive oil: 1 tbsp (15 ml / 0.5 oz)
- Lemon juice: 1 tbsp (15 ml / 0.5 oz)
- Salt and pepper to taste

Instructions:

1. Season the chicken breast with salt and pepper, sear in olive oil until golden brown, then bake for 10-12 minutes at 180°C / 350°F.
2. Cook the quinoa in salted water (100 ml / 3.5 oz) for about 15 minutes.
3. Steam or boil the broccoli for 5-7 minutes.
4. Serve the chicken with quinoa and broccoli, drizzling with lemon juice.

Nutritional Information:

- Calories: 450 kcal
- Protein: 35g
- Fat: 18g
- Yield: 400g / 14 oz
- Cooking Time: 30 minutes
- Cooking Temperature: 180°C / 350°F

Dinner: Salmon with Roasted Vegetables

Ingredients:

- Salmon fillet: 150g / 5.3 oz
- Zucchini: 100g / 3.5 oz
- Carrot: 80g / 2.8 oz
- Bell pepper: 1 (150g / 5.3 oz)
- Olive oil: 1 tbsp (15 ml / 0.5 oz)
- Salt and spices to taste

Instructions:

1. Chop the vegetables and place them in a baking dish.
2. Season with salt and spices, drizzle with olive oil.
3. Place the salmon fillet on top of the vegetables, season with salt and pepper.
4. Bake at 200°C / 400°F for about 20-25 minutes.

Nutritional Information:

- Calories: 350 kcal
- Protein: 30g
- Fat: 22g
- Yield: 480g / 17 oz
- Cooking Time: 35 minutes
- Cooking Temperature: 200°C / 400°F

Meal Plan 2

Breakfast: Buckwheat Porridge with Berries and Nuts
Ingredients:
- Buckwheat: 50g / 1.7 oz
- Water: 150 ml / 5.3 oz
- Berries (blueberries, raspberries): 50g / 1.7 oz
- Walnuts: 10g / 0.35 oz
- Honey: 1 tsp (5g / 0.17 oz)

Instructions:
1. Cook the buckwheat in water until done (about 15 minutes).
2. Mix the buckwheat with berries and sprinkle with nuts.
3. Drizzle the porridge with honey before serving.

Nutritional Information:
- Calories: 280 kcal
- Protein: 7g
- Fat: 7g
- Yield: 160g / 5.6 oz
- Cooking Time: 20 minutes
- Cooking Temperature: Medium heat

Lunch: Ratatouille with Chicken Fillet
Ingredients:
- Chicken fillet: 150g / 5.3 oz
- Eggplant: 100g / 3.5 oz
- Zucchini: 100g / 3.5 oz
- Tomato: 1 (100g / 3.5 oz)
- Olive oil: 1 tbsp (15 ml / 0.5 oz)
- Garlic: 1 clove
- Italian herbs to taste
- Salt and pepper to taste

Instructions:
1. Slice the eggplant, zucchini, and tomato into thin rounds.
2. Layer the vegetables in a baking dish, adding garlic and herbs.
3. Sear the chicken fillet in olive oil until golden brown, then place it on top of the vegetables.
4. Bake at 180°C / 350°F for about 25 minutes.

Nutritional Information:

- Calories: 350 kcal
- Protein: 28g
- Fat: 15g
- Yield: 450g / 16 oz
- Cooking Time: 40 minutes
- Cooking Temperature: 180°C / 350°F

Dinner: Tuna and Avocado Salad
Ingredients:

- Tuna in water: 100g / 3.5 oz
- Avocado: ½ (70g / 2.5 oz)
- Lettuce leaves: 50g / 1.7 oz
- Cucumber: 1 (100g / 3.5 oz)
- Olive oil: 1 tbsp (15 ml / 0.5 oz)
- Lemon juice: 1 tsp (5 ml / 0.17 oz)
- Salt and pepper to taste

Instructions:

1. Slice the avocado and cucumber, mix with the lettuce leaves.
2. Add the tuna, season with olive oil and lemon juice.
3. Toss the salad before serving.

Nutritional Information:

- Calories: 300 kcal
- Protein: 20g
- Fat: 22g
- Yield: 320g / 11.3 oz
- Cooking Time: 10 minutes
- Cooking Temperature: None required

Meal Plan 3

Breakfast: Oatmeal with Apples and Cinnamon
Ingredients:

- Oats: 50g / 1.7 oz
- Water or milk: 200 ml / 7 oz
- Apple: 1 (150g / 5.3 oz)
- Cinnamon: ½ tsp (2g / 0.07 oz)

- Honey: 1 tsp (5g / 0.17 oz)

Instructions:

1. Cook the oats in water or milk.
2. Dice the apple and add to the oatmeal with cinnamon.
3. Drizzle with honey before serving.

Nutritional Information:

- Calories: 290 kcal
- Protein: 6g
- Fat: 5g
- Yield: 250g / 8.8 oz
- Cooking Time: 15 minutes
- Cooking Temperature: Medium heat

Lunch: Fish Cakes with Mashed Potatoes

Ingredients:

- White fish fillet: 200g / 7 oz
- Potato: 150g / 5.3 oz
- Onion: 50g / 1.7 oz
- Egg: 1 (60g / 2.1 oz)
- Bread crumbs: 30g / 1 oz
- Olive oil: 1 tbsp (15 ml / 0.5 oz)
- Salt and pepper to taste

Instructions:

1. Boil the potatoes and make mashed potatoes.
2. Blend the fish fillet, onion, and egg in a blender, season, and add bread crumbs.
3. Shape the mixture into patties and fry in olive oil until golden brown.
4. Serve with mashed potatoes.

Nutritional Information:

- Calories: 400 kcal
- Protein: 25g
- Fat: 18g
- Yield: 380g / 13.4 oz
- Cooking Time: 35 minutes
- Cooking Temperature: Medium heat

Dinner: Greek Salad with Chicken
Ingredients:

- Chicken breast: 150g / 5.3 oz
- Tomatoes: 100g / 3.5 oz
- Cucumbers: 100g / 3.5 oz
- Olives: 50g / 1.7 oz
- Feta cheese: 50g / 1.7 oz
- Red onion: 30g / 1 oz
- Olive oil: 1 tbsp (15 ml / 0.5 oz)
- Oregano to taste
- Salt and pepper to taste

Instructions:

1. Grill or pan-sear the chicken breast until cooked through.
2. Dice the tomatoes, cucumbers, onion, and feta.
3. Combine all ingredients with the olives, add the chicken.
4. Dress the salad with olive oil and oregano.

Nutritional Information:

- Calories: 320 kcal
- Protein: 28g
- Fat: 20g
- Yield: 350g / 12.

Meal Plan 4

Breakfast: Avocado and Egg Toasts
Ingredients:

- Whole grain bread: 2 slices (60g / 2.1 oz)
- Avocado: ½ (70g / 2.5 oz)
- Egg: 1 (60g / 2.1 oz)
- Lemon juice: 1 tsp (5 ml / 0.17 oz)
- Salt and pepper to taste

Instructions:

1. Toast the bread in a toaster.
2. Mash the avocado with lemon juice, and add salt and pepper.
3. Boil the egg and place it on the toast topped with avocado.

- Calories: 250 kcal
- Protein: 9g
- Fat: 16g
- Yield: 190g / 6.7 oz
- Cooking Time: 10 minutes
- Cooking Temperature: Not required

Lunch: Turkey with Bulgur and Vegetables

Ingredients:

- Turkey fillet: 200g / 7 oz
- Bulgur: 50g / 1.7 oz
- Carrot: 100g / 3.5 oz
- Broccoli: 100g / 3.5 oz
- Olive oil: 1 tbsp (15 ml / 0.5 oz)
- Garlic: 1 clove
- Salt and pepper to taste

Instructions:

1. Cut the turkey into pieces and sauté in olive oil until golden brown.
2. Cook the bulgur in salted water (100 ml / 3.5 oz) for about 15 minutes.
3. Slice the carrot into strips, divide the broccoli into florets, and cook together for 5-7 minutes.
4. Serve the turkey with bulgur and vegetables.

Nutritional Information:

- Calories: 380 kcal
- Protein: 32g
- Fat: 15g
- Yield: 450g / 16 oz
- Cooking Time: 30 minutes
- Cooking Temperature: Medium heat

Dinner: Baked Cod with Vegetables

Ingredients:

- Cod fillet: 200g / 7 oz
- Zucchini: 100g / 3.5 oz
- Bell pepper: 1 (150g / 5.3 oz)
- Olive oil: 1 tbsp (15 ml / 0.5 oz)

- Lemon juice: 1 tbsp (15 ml / 0.5 oz)
- Spices (thyme, rosemary) to taste
- Salt and pepper to taste

Instructions:
1. Cut the zucchini and bell pepper into cubes.
2. Place the vegetables in a baking dish, season with salt, pepper, and spices
3. Lay the cod fillet on top, and drizzle with lemon juice.
4. Bake at 180°C / 350°F for about 20 minutes.

Nutritional Information:
- Calories: 310 kcal
- Protein: 30g
- Fat: 14g
- Yield: 450g / 16 oz
- Cooking Time: 30 minutes
- Cooking Temperature: 180°C / 350°F

Meal Plan 5

Breakfast: Banana and Spinach Smoothie
Ingredients:
- Banana: 1 (120g / 4.2 oz)
- Spinach: 50g / 1.7 oz
- Almond milk: 200 ml / 7 oz
- Chia seeds: 1 tsp (5g / 0.17 oz)

Instructions:
1. Blend the banana, spinach, almond milk, and chia seeds in a blender.
2. Pour the smoothie into a glass and serve immediately.

Nutritional Information:
- Calories: 250 kcal
- Protein: 5g
- Fat: 7g
- Yield: 350 ml / 12 oz
- Cooking Time: 5 minutes
- Cooking Temperature: Not required

Lunch: Beef Steak with Vegetable Garnish
Ingredients:

- Beef steak: 200g / 7 oz
- Green beans: 100g / 3.5 oz
- Potato: 150g / 5.3 oz
- Olive oil: 1 tbsp (15 ml / 0.5 oz)
- Salt and pepper to taste

Instructions:

1. Grill or pan-fry the steak to your desired doneness.
2. Boil the potatoes and green beans until tender.
3. Serve the steak with the vegetables, seasoning with olive oil and spices.

Nutritional Information:

- Calories: 500 kcal
- Protein: 40g
- Fat: 25g
- Yield: 450g / 16 oz
- Cooking Time: 25 minutes
- Cooking Temperature: Medium heat

Dinner: Stewed Turkey with Mushrooms and Rice
Ingredients:

- Turkey fillet: 150g / 5.3 oz
- Mushrooms (champignons): 100g / 3.5 oz
- Rice: 50g / 1.7 oz
- Olive oil: 1 tbsp (15 ml / 0.5 oz)
- Onion: 50g / 1.7 oz
- Salt and pepper to taste

Instructions:

1. Cut the turkey into cubes and sauté in olive oil until cooked.
2. Add chopped mushrooms and onion, and stew for 5-7 minutes.
3. Cook the rice in salted water (100 ml / 3.5 oz) for about 15 minutes.
4. Serve the turkey with rice.

Nutritional Information:

- Calories: 380 kcal
- Protein: 28g
- Fat: 14g
- Yield: 350g / 12.3 oz

- Cooking Time: 35 minutes
- Cooking Temperature: Medium heat

Meal Plan 6

Breakfast: Spelt Porridge with Nuts and Dried Fruits
Ingredients:
- Spelt: 50g / 1.7 oz
- Water: 200 ml / 7 oz
- Walnuts: 10g / 0.35 oz
- Dried fruits (apricots, raisins): 30g / 1 oz
- Honey: 1 tsp (5g / 0.17 oz)

Instructions:
1. Cook the spelt in water until done (about 20 minutes).
2. Add chopped nuts and dried fruits.
3. Drizzle with honey before serving.

Nutritional Information:
- Calories: 300 kcal
- Protein: 7g
- Fat: 9g
- Yield: 180g / 6.3 oz
- Cooking Time: 25 minutes
- Cooking Temperature: Medium heat

Lunch: Quinoa Salad with Avocado and Beans
Ingredients:
- Quinoa: 50g / 1.7 oz
- Red beans: 100g / 3.5 oz
- Avocado: ½ (70g / 2.5 oz)
- Cherry tomatoes: 50g / 1.7 oz
- Olive oil: 1 tbsp (15 ml / 0.5 oz)
- Lemon juice: 1 tsp (5 ml / 0.17 oz)
- Salt and pepper to taste

Instructions:
1. Cook the quinoa in salted water (100 ml / 3.5 oz) for about 15 minutes.
2. Slice the avocado and cherry tomatoes.
3. Mix all the ingredients, add beans, and dress with olive oil and lemon juice.

Nutritional Information:

- Calories: 330 kcal
- Protein: 9g
- Fat: 18g
- Yield: 250g / 8.8 oz
- Cooking Time: 20 minutes
- Cooking Temperature: Not required

Dinner: Stewed Chicken with Vegetables

Ingredients:

- Chicken fillet: 200g / 7 oz
- Carrot: 100g / 3.5 oz
- Zucchini: 100g / 3.5 oz
- Onion: 50g / 1.7 oz
- Garlic: 1 clove
- Olive oil: 1 tbsp (15 ml / 0.5 oz)
- Salt and pepper to taste

Instructions:

1. Cut the chicken into cubes and sauté in olive oil until golden brown.
2. Slice the carrot, zucchini, and onion, and add them to the chicken.
3. Add garlic and spices, and stew for 20 minutes on low heat.

Nutritional Information:

- Calories: 350 kcal
- Protein: 30g
- Fat: 15g
- Yield: 400g / 14 oz
- Cooking Time: 35 minutes
- Cooking Temperature: Medium heat

Meal Plan 7

Breakfast: Buckwheat Porridge with Pumpkin and Honey

Ingredients:

- Buckwheat: 50 g / 1.7 oz
- Pumpkin: 100 g / 3.5 oz
- Water: 200 ml / 7 oz

- Honey: 1 tsp (5 g / 0.17 oz)
- Cinnamon to taste

Cooking Process:
1. Boil the buckwheat in water until cooked.
2. Dice the pumpkin, add to the buckwheat, and cook for another 10 minutes.
3. Drizzle with honey and sprinkle with cinnamon before serving.

Calories: 260 kcal
Proteins: 5 g
Fats: 4 g
Final Dish Yield: 250 g / 8.8 oz
Cooking Time: 20 minutes
Cooking Temperature: Medium heat

Lunch: Chicken Meatballs with Vegetable Stew

Ingredients:
- Ground chicken: 200 g / 7 oz
- Zucchini: 100 g / 3.5 oz
- Carrot: 100 g / 3.5 oz
- Tomatoes: 100 g / 3.5 oz
- Onion: 50 g / 1.7 oz
- Olive oil: 1 tbsp (15 ml / 0.5 oz)
- Garlic: 1 clove
- Salt and pepper to taste

Cooking Process:
1. Form meatballs from the ground chicken.
2. Fry them in olive oil until golden brown.
3. Dice the vegetables, add to the meatballs, and simmer on low heat for 20 minutes.

Calories: 370 kcal
Proteins: 28 g
Fats: 18 g
Final Dish Yield: 400 g / 14 oz
Cooking Time: 35 minutes
Cooking Temperature: Medium heat

Dinner: Steamed Salmon with Broccoli
Ingredients:

- Salmon fillet: 200 g / 7 oz
- Broccoli: 100 g / 3.5 oz
- Lemon juice: 1 tbsp (15 ml / 0.5 oz)
- Salt and pepper to taste

Cooking Process:

1. Place the salmon in a steamer, sprinkle with salt and pepper.
2. Arrange the broccoli next to the salmon.
3. Steam for 15 minutes, then drizzle with lemon juice before serving.

Calories: 320 kcal
Proteins: 30 g
Fats: 20 g
Final Dish Yield: 300 g / 10.6 oz
Cooking Time: 20 minutes
Cooking Temperature: Medium heat

Meal Plan 8

Breakfast: Oat Pancake with Cottage Cheese and Berries
Ingredients:

- Oats: 50 g / 1.7 oz
- Egg: 1 pc (60 g / 2.1 oz)
- Milk: 50 ml / 1.7 oz
- Cottage cheese: 100 g / 3.5 oz
- Berries (raspberries, blueberries): 50 g / 1.7 oz
- Honey: 1 tsp (5 g / 0.17 oz)

Cooking Process:

1. Mix the oats, egg, and milk, and fry on a non-stick skillet.
2. Place the oat pancake on a plate, spread with cottage cheese, and add berries.
3. Drizzle with honey before serving.

Calories: 290 kcal
Proteins: 15 g
Fats: 9 g
Final Dish Yield: 250 g / 8.8 oz

Cooking Time: 15 minutes
Cooking Temperature: Medium heat

Lunch: Stewed Beef with Vegetables and Rice

Ingredients:

- Beef (lean): 200 g / 7 oz
- Carrot: 100 g / 3.5 oz
- Onion: 50 g / 1.7 oz
- Sweet pepper: 100 g / 3.5 oz
- Rice: 50 g / 1.7 oz
- Olive oil: 1 tbsp (15 ml / 0.5 oz)
- Garlic: 1 clove
- Salt and pepper to taste

Cooking Process:

1. Dice the beef, fry in olive oil until done.
2. Add the diced vegetables and garlic, and stew on low heat for 20 minutes
3. Cook the rice in salted water (100 ml / 3.5 oz) for about 15 minutes.
4. Serve the beef with vegetables and rice.

Calories: 420 kcal

Proteins: 30 g

Fats: 20 g

Final Dish Yield: 400 g / 14 oz

Cooking Time: 35 minutes

Cooking Temperature: Medium heat

Dinner: Chicken and Pineapple Salad

Ingredients:

- Chicken breast: 150 g / 5.3 oz
- Pineapple (fresh or canned): 100 g / 3.5 oz
- Lettuce leaves: 50 g / 1.7 oz
- Nuts (walnuts or cashews): 20 g / 0.7 oz
- Olive oil: 1 tbsp (15 ml / 0.5 oz)
- Salt and pepper to taste

Cooking Process:

1. Grill or pan-fry the chicken breast until done.
2. Dice the pineapple, mix with lettuce leaves and nuts.
3. Add the chicken, and drizzle with olive oil before serving.

Calories: 320 kcal
Proteins: 25 g
Fats: 18 g
Final Dish Yield: 300 g / 10.6 oz
Cooking Time: 20 minutes
Cooking Temperature: No heat required

Meal Plan 9

Breakfast: Yogurt with Muesli and Berries
Ingredients:

- Natural yogurt: 150 g / 5.3 oz
- Muesli: 50 g / 1.7 oz
- Berries (strawberries, blueberries): 50 g / 1.7 oz
- Honey: 1 tsp (5 g / 0.17 oz)

Cooking Process:

1. In a bowl, mix yogurt with muesli and berries.
2. Drizzle with honey before serving.

Calories: 220 kcal
Proteins: 10 g
Fats: 5 g
Final Dish Yield: 250 g / 8.8 oz
Cooking Time: 5 minutes
Cooking Temperature: No heat required

Lunch: Pasta with Chicken and Vegetables
Ingredients:

- Pasta (spaghetti or penne): 100 g / 3.5 oz
- Chicken fillet: 150 g / 5.3 oz
- Tomatoes: 100 g / 3.5 oz
- Zucchini: 100 g / 3.5 oz
- Garlic: 1 clove
- Olive oil: 1 tbsp (15 ml / 0.5 oz)
- Salt and pepper to taste

Cooking Process:

1. Boil the pasta in salted water until done.
2. Dice the chicken fillet, fry in olive oil with garlic.

3. Add the diced tomatoes and zucchini, and stew for 10 minutes.
4. Mix the pasta with the chicken and vegetables before serving.

Calories: 430 kcal
Proteins: 25 g
Fats: 15 g
Final Dish Yield: 400 g / 14 oz
Cooking Time: 25 minutes
Cooking Temperature: Medium heat

Dinner: Omelet with Mushrooms and Spinach

Ingredients:

- Eggs: 2 pcs (120 g / 4.2 oz)
- Mushrooms (champignons): 100 g / 3.5 oz
- Spinach: 50 g / 1.7 oz
- Milk: 50 ml / 1.7 oz
- Olive oil: 1 tbsp (15 ml / 0.5 oz)
- Salt and pepper to taste

Cooking Process:

1. Dice the mushrooms and spinach.
2. Fry the mushrooms in olive oil, then add the spinach.
3. Beat the eggs with milk, pour into the pan, and cook the omelet until done.

Calories: 280 kcal
Proteins: 18 g
Fats: 20 g
Final Dish Yield: 250 g / 8.8 oz
Cooking Time: 15 minutes
Cooking Temperature: Medium heat

Meal Plan 10

Breakfast: Pancakes with Oat Bran and Yogurt

Ingredients:

- Oat bran: 50 g / 1.7 oz
- Milk: 100 ml / 3.5 oz
- Egg: 1 pc (60 g / 2.1 oz)
- Natural yogurt: 100 g / 3.5 oz
- Honey: 1 tsp (5 g / 0.17 oz)

Cooking Process:

1. Mix the oat bran, milk, and egg, and cook pancakes on a non-stick skillet.
2. Serve the pancakes with yogurt and honey.

Calories: 290 kcal

Proteins: 10 g

Fats: 9 g

Final Dish Yield: 250 g / 8.8 oz

Cooking Time: 15 minutes

Cooking Temperature: Medium heat

Lunch: Turkey with Quinoa and Vegetables

Ingredients:

- Turkey fillet: 200 g / 7 oz
- Quinoa: 50 g / 1.7 oz
- Carrot: 100 g / 3.5 oz
- Green beans: 100 g / 3.5 oz
- Olive oil: 1 tbsp (15 ml / 0.5 oz)
- Salt and pepper to taste

Cooking Process:

1. Cut the turkey into cubes and sauté in olive oil until cooked.
2. Boil the quinoa in salted water (100 ml / 3.5 oz) for about 15 minutes.
3. Slice the carrot, add it to the turkey, and simmer for 10 minutes.
4. Serve the turkey with quinoa and vegetables.

Calories: 380 kcal

Proteins: 28 g

Fats: 14 g

Total Dish Weight: 400 g / 14 oz

Cooking Time: 30 minutes

Cooking Temperature: Medium heat

Dinner: Fish with Potatoes and Vegetables

Ingredients:

- Fish fillet (cod, pike): 200 g / 7 oz
- Potato: 100 g / 3.5 oz
- Zucchini: 100 g / 3.5 oz
- Carrot: 100 g / 3.5 oz
- Olive oil: 1 tbsp (15 ml / 0.5 oz)

- Lemon juice: 1 tbsp (15 ml / 0.5 oz)
- Salt and pepper to taste

Cooking Process:

1. Cut the potatoes, zucchini, and carrot into cubes, and bake in the oven for 20 minutes at 180°C / 350°F.
2. Drizzle the fish fillet with lemon juice, add salt and pepper, and place it on top of the vegetables.
3. Bake everything together for another 10 minutes.

Calories*: 340 kcal

Proteins*: 30 g

**Fat*s*: 15 g

Total Dish Weight*: 400 g / 14 oz

Cooking Time*: 30 minutes

Cooking Temperature*: 180°C / 350°F

Chapter 6: Meat Dishes and Burgers, 13 Recipes

Meat dishes and burgers can be included in the diet even when losing weight, if you use lean meats, the right additives, and whole grain buns. **Burger and cheeseburger recipes** contain less fat and calories but are rich in protein and fiber, making them suitable for healthy eating and weight maintenance.

1. Beef Steaks with Grilled Vegetables

Ingredients:

- 200 g beef steak (e.g., fillet or tenderloin)
- 1 bell pepper
- 1 zucchini
- 1 small eggplant
- 1 tsp olive oil
- Spices to taste (salt, pepper, rosemary, thyme)

Preparation:

1. Cut the bell pepper, zucchini, and eggplant into large pieces.
2. Mix the olive oil with spices and rub this mixture onto the steak.
3. Heat the grill or grill pan and sear the steak to the desired level of doneness (3-4 minutes on each side for medium rare).
4. Place the vegetables on the grill and cook until soft.
5. Serve the steak with the vegetables, garnished with herbs.

2. Beef Meatballs in Tomato Sauce

Ingredients:

- 300 g lean ground beef
- 1 egg
- 1 onion, finely chopped
- 2 garlic cloves, minced
- 400 g canned tomatoes (unsweetened, unsalted)
- 1 tbsp olive oil
- Spices to taste (salt, pepper, basil, oregano)

Preparation:
1. In a bowl, mix the ground beef, egg, half of the onion, and garlic, then add salt and pepper. Form small meatballs.
2. Sear the meatballs in a dry pan until browned, then remove from the pan.
3. In the same pan, sauté the remaining onion and garlic in olive oil until soft, then add the canned tomatoes and spices.
4. Place the meatballs into the sauce, cover, and simmer over low heat for 15-20 minutes.
5. Serve with herbs and whole grain pasta or quinoa.

3. Beef Stew with Vegetables

Ingredients:
- 200 g beef (fillet or tenderloin)
- 200 g broccoli
- 100 g mushrooms
- 1 onion
- 1 tsp low-sodium soy sauce
- 1 tsp sesame oil
- Spices to taste (ginger, garlic, black pepper)

Preparation:
1. Slice the beef into thin strips, the onion into half rings, and the mushrooms into slices.
2. Sear the beef in sesame oil until golden brown, then add the onion and mushrooms.
3. When the mushrooms start to reduce in volume, add the broccoli and soy sauce, and mix well.
4. Cook everything together for another 5-7 minutes until the broccoli softens
5. Serve the dish sprinkled with sesame seeds.

4. Beef with Broccoli and Mushrooms

Ingredients:
- 200 g beef (fillet or tenderloin)

- 200 g broccoli
- 100 g mushrooms
- 1 onion
- 1 tsp low-sodium soy sauce
- 1 tsp sesame oil
- Spices to taste (ginger, garlic, black pepper)

Preparation:

1. Slice the beef into thin strips, the onion into half rings, and the mushrooms into slices.
2. Sear the beef in sesame oil until golden brown, then add the onion and mushrooms.
3. When the mushrooms start to reduce in volume, add the broccoli and soy sauce, and mix well.
4. Cook everything together for another 5-7 minutes until the broccoli softens.
5. Serve the dish sprinkled with sesame seeds.

5. Beef and Quinoa Salad

Ingredients:

- 150 g beef steak (fillet)
- 50 g cooked quinoa
- 1 cucumber
- 1 bell pepper
- Spinach or lettuce leaves
- 1 tbsp olive oil
- 1 tsp balsamic vinegar
- Spices to taste (salt, pepper, dried garlic)

Preparation:

1. Grill or pan-sear the steak to your desired doneness, then slice it thinly.
2. Cut the cucumber and bell pepper into cubes.
3. Place spinach in a bowl, add the chopped vegetables, quinoa, and beef slices.

4. Dress the salad with a mixture of olive oil and balsamic vinegar, and add spices to taste.
5. Toss and serve immediately.

6. Lean Beef Burger with Greek Yogurt

Ingredients:

- 150 g lean ground beef
- 1 whole-grain bun
- 1 tbsp Greek yogurt
- Lettuce leaves
- 1 slice of tomato
- 1/2 avocado (optional)
- Spices to taste (salt, pepper, garlic, paprika)

Preparation:

1. Mix the ground beef with spices and shape it into a patty.
2. Cook the patty in a non-stick pan or bake it in the oven.
3. Cut the bun in half and lightly toast it in a toaster.
4. Spread Greek yogurt on the bottom half of the bun.
5. Place the patty on the bun, add lettuce leaves, a slice of tomato, and avocado pieces.
6. Cover with the top half of the bun and serve.

7. Chicken Breast Burger with Greens

Ingredients:

- 150 g chicken fillet
- 1 whole-grain bun
- Spinach or lettuce leaves
- 1 slice of cucumber
- 1 tsp mustard
- 1 tbsp low-fat natural yogurt
- Spices to taste (salt, pepper, garlic, thyme)

Preparation:
1. Mince the chicken fillet, add spices, and shape it into a patty.
2. Cook the patty on a grill or in a non-stick pan.
3. Cut the bun in half and lightly toast it in a toaster.
4. Mix the yogurt with mustard and spread it on the bottom half of the bun.
5. Place the patty on the bun, add spinach and a slice of cucumber.
6. Cover with the other half of the bun and serve.

8. Spiced Turkey Burger

Ingredients:
- 150 g turkey (ground)
- 1 whole-grain bun
- 1 slice of low-fat cheese (e.g., mozzarella)
- 1 tomato
- Lettuce leaves
- 1 tbsp hummus
- Spices to taste (turmeric, coriander, cumin, paprika)

Preparation:
1. Mix the ground turkey with spices and shape it into a patty.
2. Cook the patty in a pan or bake it in the oven.
3. Cut the bun in half and lightly toast it in a toaster.
4. Spread hummus on the bottom half of the bun.
5. Place the patty, add a slice of cheese, tomato, and lettuce.
6. Cover with the top half of the bun and serve.

9. Beef Burger with Mushrooms and Spinach

Ingredients:
- 150 g lean ground beef
- 1 whole-grain bun
- 100 g mushrooms
- 1 tbsp low fat natural yogurt
- Spinach leaves

- Spices to taste (salt, pepper, garlic, oregano)

Preparation:

1. Slice the mushrooms and sauté them in a pan without oil until golden brown.
2. Mix the ground beef with spices and shape it into a patty. Cook the patty until done.
3. Cut the bun in half and lightly toast it in a toaster.
4. Spread yogurt on the bottom half of the bun, then layer with the patty, sautéed mushrooms, and spinach leaves.
5. Cover with the top half of the bun and serve.

10. Mexican Beef Burger with Avocado

Ingredients:

- 150 g lean ground beef
- 1 whole-grain bun
- 1/2 avocado
- 1 tbsp salsa (tomato sauce)
- Lettuce leaves
- 1 tsp lemon juice
- Spices to taste (chili, coriander, cumin, black pepper)

Preparation:

1. Mix the ground beef with spices and shape it into a patty.
2. Cook the patty on a grill or in a pan until done.
3. Mash the avocado with lemon juice and a pinch of salt.
4. Cut the bun in half and lightly toast it in a toaster.
5. Spread the mashed avocado on the bottom half of the bun, then add the patty, salsa, and lettuce.
6. Cover with the top half of the bun and serve.

11. Turkey Burger with Avocado

Ingredients:

- 200 g turkey fillet (or chicken breast)

- 1 avocado
- 1 whole-grain bun
- Lettuce leaves
- 1 slice of tomato
- 1 slice of onion (optional)
- 1 tsp olive oil
- Spices to taste (black pepper, garlic, paprika)

Preparation:

1. Mince the turkey fillet and add spices to taste.
2. Shape the ground turkey into a patty and cook it in a pan with minimal olive oil or bake in the oven until done.
3. Cut the bun in half and lightly toast it in a pan or toaster.
4. Mash half of the avocado with a fork and spread it on one half of the bun.
5. Place the turkey patty on top, then add lettuce leaves, a slice of tomato, and onion.
6. Cover with the top half of the bun and serve.

2. Chicken Cheeseburger with Yogurt Sauce

Ingredients:

- 200 g chicken fillet
- 1 slice of low-fat cheese (e.g., mozzarella or Gouda)
- 1 whole-grain bun
- Lettuce leaves
- 1 slice of cucumber
- 2 tbsp Greek yogurt
- 1 tsp mustard
- 1 tsp lemon juice
- Spices to taste (salt, pepper, paprika)

Preparation:

1. Mince the chicken fillet and add spices. Shape the mixture into a patty.
2. Cook the patty on a dry pan or grill until done. A few minutes before it's finished, place the cheese slice on the patty to melt.

3. Cut the bun in half and toast it in the toaster.
4. Mix Greek yogurt with mustard and lemon juice to make the sauce.
5. Spread the sauce on both halves of the bun.
6. Place the patty with melted cheese on the bun, add lettuce leaves and a slice of cucumber.
7. Cover with the top half of the bun and serve.

13. Vegetarian Burger with Quinoa and Black Beans

Ingredients:

- 100 g cooked quinoa
- 100 g black beans (canned or cooked)
- 1 carrot, grated
- 1 egg
- 1 whole-grain bun
- Lettuce leaves
- 1 slice of tomato
- 1 tsp olive oil
- Spices to taste (cumin, garlic, paprika, black pepper)

Preparation:

1. In a bowl, mash the black beans with a fork, leaving some texture.
2. Add cooked quinoa, grated carrot, egg, and spices. Mix well.
3. Shape the mixture into patties and fry them in a pan with a small amount of olive oil until golden brown.
4. Toast the bun in the toaster.
5. Place a lettuce leaf on the bottom half of the bun, add the patty, then a slice of tomato, and cover with the top half of the bun. Serve immediately.

Chapter 7: Delicious Snacks for Healthy Eating

Healthy snacks for weight loss can be both tasty and beneficial. They help maintain a feeling of fullness between main meals, provide energy, and prevent overeating throughout the day. Here are some snack options you can include in your diet:

1. **Nuts and Seeds**

   - **Portion:** 30 g (1 oz)

   - **Calories:** About 160-200 kcal

   - **Benefits:** Nuts and seeds are rich in healthy fats, proteins, and fiber. They help maintain energy levels and stabilize blood sugar.

2. **Yogurt with Fruit**

   - **Portion:** 150 g (5.3 oz)

   - **Calories:** About 100-150 kcal (depending on the fat content of the yogurt)

   - **Benefits:** Yogurt contains probiotics that support gut health, and fruits add natural sweetness and vitamins.

3. **Carrot Sticks with Hummus**

   - **Portion:** 100 g of carrots + 50 g of hummus (3.5 oz of carrots + 1.7 oz of hummus)

   - **Calories:** About 100-120 kcal

   - **Benefits:** This snack combines fiber and vitamins from carrots with plant-based protein from hummus.

4. **Apple with Almond Butter**

   - **Portion:** 1 apple (150 g / 5.3 oz) + 1 tbsp of almond butter (15 g / 0.5 oz)

- o **Calories:** About 200 kcal

- o **Benefits:** Apples are rich in fiber, and almond butter contains healthy fats and proteins.

5. **Vegetable Chips**

- o **Portion:** 30 g (1 oz)

- o **Calories:** About 50-80 kcal

- o **Benefits:** Vegetable chips made from beets, carrots, or zucchini are a low-calorie alternative to regular potato chips, rich in fiber.

6. **Greek Yogurt with Berries**

- o **Portion:** 150 g of Greek yogurt + 50 g of berries (5.3 oz of yogurt + 1.7 oz of berries)

- o **Calories:** About 100-120 kcal

- o **Benefits:** Greek yogurt contains more protein than regular yogurt, and berries add antioxidants and fiber.

7. **Celery with Peanut Butter**

- o **Portion:** 2-3 celery stalks + 1 tbsp of peanut butter (40 g / 1.4 oz of celery + 15 g / 0.5 oz of butter)

- o **Calories:** About 150 kcal

- o **Benefits:** Celery is low in calories but high in fiber, and peanut butter adds flavor and healthy fats.

8. **Protein Bar**

- o **Portion:** 1 bar (about 50 g / 1.7 oz)

- o **Calories:** About 200 kcal

- o **Benefits:** Protein bars are great for satisfying hunger and maintaining protein levels, which is important for preserving muscle mass during weight loss.

9. **Boiled Eggs**

- o **Portion:** 2 eggs (100 g / 3.5 oz)

- o **Calories:** About 140 kcal

- o **Benefits:** Eggs are rich in protein and contain all the essential amino acids, making them an ideal snack for maintaining energy.

10. **Smoothie with Greens and Fruits**

- **Portion:** 250 ml (1 cup / 8.5 oz)

- **Calories:** About 150-200 kcal

- **Benefits:** Smoothies made with greens (like spinach) and fruits (like bananas or berries) are rich in vitamins, minerals, and fiber.

These snacks will help you control your appetite and avoid overeating, providing you with the necessary nutrients to maintain health and achieve successful weight loss.

Chapter 8: Can Delicious and Sweet Desserts Be Low-Calorie and Healthy?

Yes, delicious and sweet desserts can be low-calorie and healthy! The key is in choosing the right ingredients and approach to preparation. Here are several ways to create such desserts:

1. **Using Natural Sugar Substitutes**: Instead of sugar, you can use natural sweeteners like stevia, erythritol, or a small amount of maple syrup. These provide sweetness without the extra calories.

2. **Fruit as a Base**: Fruits like berries, bananas, or apples contain natural sweetness and are packed with beneficial nutrients. They can be the base for fruit salads, smoothies, baked desserts, or sorbets.

3. **Greek Yogurt**: This product is an excellent alternative to heavy cream and butter. It adds a creamy texture to desserts like cheesecakes or mousses while remaining low in calories and rich in protein.

4. **Oats and Nuts**: Adding oats and nuts to desserts like muffins or cookies increases fiber and healthy fats, making them more filling and nutritious.

5. **Cocoa Powder**: Unsweetened cocoa powder is a great way to add rich chocolate flavor to desserts without adding extra calories. It can be used in making low-calorie brownies, chocolate puddings, or mousses.

6. **Avocado**: Avocado can be an excellent base for chocolate mousse or cake frosting. It gives a creamy texture to the dish and is rich in healthy fats that help absorb vitamins.

7. **Frozen Desserts**: Sorbets, frozen yogurts, and fruit popsicles are great low-calorie alternatives to ice cream. They can be made at home from fresh fruits and berries with minimal added sweeteners.

Examples of Healthy Desserts:

- **Berry Sorbet**: A blend of frozen berries and a bit of stevia is a tasty and refreshing dessert without sugar and extra calories.

- **Greek Yogurt Cheesecake**: A light and low-calorie version of the classic dessert using Greek yogurt instead of heavy cream.

- **Avocado Chocolate Mousse**: A creamy and rich dessert easily made by blending avocado with cocoa powder and a small amount of honey or maple syrup.

These desserts can be enjoyed without the fear of gaining weight.

30 Low-Calorie and Healthy Desserts

This section will include 30 low-calorie and healthy desserts. Each recipe will contain the necessary ingredients, the entire preparation process, the yield of the finished dessert, the preparation time, and the calorie content.

Recipe 1: Avocado Chocolate Mousse
Ingredients:
- Ripe avocados – 2 (about 400 g or 0.88 lb)
- Cocoa powder (unsweetened) – 40 g (0.09 lb)
- Honey or maple syrup – 60 g (0.13 lb)
- Vanilla extract – 1 teaspoon (about 5 ml or 0.17 oz)
- Coconut milk – 100 ml (3.38 oz)

Preparation Process:
1. Cut the avocados in half, remove the pit, and scoop out the flesh with a spoon.
2. Blend the avocado flesh in a blender or food processor until smooth.
3. Add the cocoa powder, honey or maple syrup, vanilla extract, and coconut milk.
4. Blend until you achieve a smooth, creamy consistency.
5. Pour the mousse into serving cups or bowls and refrigerate for at least 30 minutes to allow it to set slightly.
6. Before serving, you can garnish with berries, nuts, or dark chocolate pieces.

Yield:
- 500 g (1.1 lb)

Preparation Time:
- About 15 minutes + 30 minutes for chilling

Calories:
- Approximately 180 kcal per serving (if divided into 4 servings)

Recipe 2: Berry Chia Pudding with Coconut Milk

Ingredients:
- 3 tablespoons chia seeds
- 200 ml coconut milk (or almond milk)
- 1 tablespoon honey or maple syrup (optional)
- 100 g fresh berries (raspberries, blueberries, strawberries)
- 1 teaspoon vanilla extract
- Almond flakes or shredded coconut for garnish

Instructions:
1. In a bowl, mix chia seeds, coconut milk, and vanilla extract. Add honey or syrup if desired.
2. Stir well to prevent the chia seeds from clumping, and leave in the refrigerator for at least 4 hours, preferably overnight.
3. Once the pudding has thickened, divide it into glasses or cups.
4. Top with fresh berries and sprinkle with almond flakes or shredded coconut.
5. Serve chilled.

Nutritional Value (per serving):
- Calories: approximately 250 kcal
- Protein: 6 g
- Fat: 18 g
- Carbohydrates: 20 g

Recipe 3: Banana Oatmeal Cookies

Ingredients:
- Oats – 150 g (0.33 lb)
- Ripe bananas – 2 (about 250 g or 0.55 lb)
- Honey – 30 g (0.07 lb)
- Cinnamon – 1 teaspoon (about 5 g or 0.01 lb)

Preparation Process:
1. Preheat the oven to 180°C (350°F).
2. Mash the bananas with a fork until they reach a puree consistency.
3. In a bowl, mix the oats, banana puree, honey, and cinnamon.

4. Form small cookies and place them on a baking sheet lined with parchment paper.
5. Bake for 15-20 minutes until golden brown.

Yield:
- 300 g (0.66 lb)

Preparation Time:
- About 30 minutes

Calories:
- Approximately 100 kcal per cookie (if divided into 10 cookies)

Recipe 4: Greek Yogurt Cheesecake

Ingredients:
- Greek yogurt – 500 g (1.1 lb)
- Honey or maple syrup – 60 g (0.13 lb)
- Gelatin – 10 g (0.02 lb)
- Water (for gelatin) – 50 ml (1.7 oz)
- Vanilla extract – 1 teaspoon (about 5 ml or 0.17 oz)
- Strawberries or other berries for decoration – 150 g (0.33 lb)

Preparation Process:
1. Soak the gelatin in cold water and let it bloom for 5 minutes.
2. In a bowl, mix Greek yogurt, honey, and vanilla extract.
3. Melt the bloomed gelatin over a double boiler and add it to the yogurt mixture, stirring thoroughly.
4. Transfer the mixture into a mold and refrigerate for 3-4 hours until fully set.
5. Before serving, decorate the cheesecake with fresh berries.

Yield:
- 700 g (1.54 lb)

Preparation Time:
- About 20 minutes + 3-4 hours to set

Calories:
- Approximately 150 kcal per serving (if divided into 6 servings)

Recipe 5: Cottage Cheese and Berry Pie

Ingredients:
- Fat-free cottage cheese – 300 g (0.66 lb)
- Eggs – 2
- Oats – 100 g (0.22 lb)

- Honey – 40 g (0.09 lb)
- Berries (raspberries, blueberries) – 200 g (0.44 lb)
- Vanilla extract – 1 teaspoon (about 5 ml or 0.17 oz)

Preparation Process:
1. Preheat the oven to 180°C (350°F).
2. In a bowl, mix oats with honey and one egg. Spread the mixture in a baking dish to form the pie crust.
3. In another bowl, mix cottage cheese, the remaining egg, and vanilla extract.
4. Pour the cottage cheese mixture over the oat crust and evenly distribute the berries on top.
5. Bake for 25-30 minutes until golden brown.

Yield:
- 600 g (1.32 lb)

Preparation Time:
- About 40 minutes

Calories:
- Approximately 150 kcal per serving (if divided into 6 servings)

Recipe 6: Almond Coconut Balls

Ingredients:
- Almonds – 200 g (0.44 lb)
- Pitted dates – 150 g (0.33 lb)
- Shredded coconut – 50 g (0.11 lb)
- Cocoa powder (unsweetened) – 20 g (0.04 lb)

Preparation Process:
1. Soak the dates in warm water for 10 minutes, then drain.
2. Blend the almonds into fine crumbs in a blender.
3. Add dates, cocoa powder, and half of the shredded coconut. Blend until a sticky mixture forms.
4. Roll the mixture into small balls and coat them with the remaining shredded coconut.
5. Refrigerate the balls for 30 minutes to set.

Yield:
- 400 g (0.88 lb)

Preparation Time:
- About 20 minutes + 30 minutes for setting

Calories:

- Approximately 120 kcal per ball (if divided into 10 balls)

Recipe 7: Pumpkin Puree with Cinnamon
Ingredients:
- Pumpkin – 500 g (1.1 lb)
- Cinnamon – 1 teaspoon (about 5 g or 0.01 lb)
- Honey or maple syrup – 30 g (0.07 lb)

Preparation Process:
1. Peel and dice the pumpkin.
2. Boil the pumpkin in a small amount of water until tender (about 15 minutes).
3. Drain the water and mash the pumpkin into a puree.
4. Add honey and cinnamon, and mix well.
5. Serve warm or chilled.

Yield:
- 500 g (1.1 lb)

Preparation Time:
- About 20 minutes

Calories:
- Approximately 80 kcal per serving (if divided into 4 servings)

Recipe 8: Apple Chips
Ingredients:
- Apples – 3 (about 400 g or 0.88 lb)
- Cinnamon – 1 teaspoon (about 5 g or 0.01 lb)

Preparation Process:
1. Preheat the oven to 100°C (210°F).
2. Slice the apples thinly and remove the core.
3. Place the slices on a baking sheet lined with parchment paper and sprinkle with cinnamon.
4. Bake the apples in the oven for 1.5-2 hours until they are crispy.

Yield:
- 100 g (0.22 lb)

Preparation Time:
- About 2 hours

Calories:
- Approximately 50 kcal per 100 g (if divided into 4 servings)

Recipe 9: Banana Strawberry Smoothie
Ingredients:
- Banana – 1 (about 120 g or 0.26 lb)
- Strawberries – 200 g (0.44 lb)
- Kefir or yogurt – 150 ml (5 oz)
- Ice – 5-6 cubes

Preparation Process:
1. Slice the banana and strawberries into pieces.
2. In a blender, combine the banana, strawberries, kefir, and ice. Blend until smooth.
3. Pour the smoothie into a glass and serve immediately.

Yield:
- 450 ml (about 15 oz)

Preparation Time:
- About 5 minutes

Calories:
- Approximately 100 kcal per serving (if divided into 2 servings)

Recipe 10: Carrot Pudding
Ingredients:
- Carrots – 300 g (0.66 lb)
- Skim milk – 200 ml (6.76 oz)
- Cinnamon – 1 teaspoon (about 5 g or 0.01 lb)
- Honey – 30 g (0.07 lb)

Preparation Process:
1. Peel and grate the carrots.
2. In a saucepan, heat the milk, add the carrots, and cook over low heat for about 15 minutes until tender.
3. Add honey and cinnamon, stir, and cook for another 5 minutes.
4. Remove from heat and divide into molds.
5. Chill the pudding before serving.

Yield:
- 500 g (1.1 lb)

Preparation Time:
- About 30 minutes

Calories:

- Approximately 120 kcal per serving (if divided into 4 servings)

Recipe 11: Avocado Chocolate Mousse

Ingredients:

- Ripe avocados – 2 (about 400 g or 0.88 lb)
- Unsweetened cocoa powder – 50 g (0.11 lb)
- Honey or maple syrup – 50 g (0.11 lb)
- Vanilla extract – 1 teaspoon (about 5 ml or 0.17 oz)
- Almond milk – 50 ml (1.69 oz)

Preparation Process:

1. Peel the avocados and remove the pits.
2. In a blender, combine avocados, cocoa powder, honey, vanilla extract, and almond milk until smooth.
3. Divide the mousse into serving cups and chill for 30 minutes before serving.

Yield:

- 500 g (1.1 lb)

Preparation Time:

- About 10 minutes + 30 minutes to chill

Calories:

- Approximately 150 kcal per serving (if divided into 4 servings)

Recipe 12: Berry Sorbet

Ingredients:

- Mixed berries (raspberries, blueberries, strawberries) – 400 g (0.88 lb)
- Honey or maple syrup – 40 g (0.09 lb)
- Lemon juice – 2 tablespoons (about 30 ml or 1 oz)

Preparation Process:

1. Freeze the berries if they are fresh.
2. In a blender, blend the frozen berries with honey and lemon juice until smooth.
3. Transfer the sorbet to a container and freeze for 1-2 hours until fully set.

Yield:

- 500 g (1.1 lb)

Preparation Time:

- About 10 minutes + 1-2 hours to freeze

Calories:

- Approximately 60 kcal per serving (if divided into 5 servings)

Recipe 13: Banana Ice Cream

Ingredients:

- Ripe bananas – 3 (about 360 g or 0.8 lb)
- Vanilla extract – 1 teaspoon (about 5 ml or 0.17 oz)
- Shredded coconut – 20 g (0.04 lb) (optional)

Preparation Process:

1. Slice the bananas and freeze them.
2. In a blender, process the frozen bananas with vanilla extract until creamy
3. Optionally, add shredded coconut and mix.
4. Serve immediately or freeze for 30 minutes for a firmer texture.

Yield:

- 400 g (0.88 lb)

Preparation Time:

- About 5 minutes + freezing time

Calories:

- Approximately 90 kcal per serving (if divided into 4 servings)

Recipe 14: Nut Bars with Honey

Ingredients:

- Oats – 100 g (0.22 lb)
- Mixed nuts (almonds, walnuts, cashews) – 100 g (0.22 lb)
- Honey – 60 g (0.13 lb)
- Coconut oil – 30 g (0.07 lb)

Preparation Process:

1. Preheat the oven to 180°C (350°F).
2. In a bowl, mix oats and chopped nuts.
3. In a saucepan, melt honey and coconut oil, then add to the oat mixture.
4. Spread the mixture on a baking sheet and press down evenly.
5. Bake for 15 minutes until golden brown.
6. Cool and cut into bars.

Yield:

- 300 g (0.66 lb)

Preparation Time:

- About 20 minutes

Calories:

- Approximately 120 kcal per bar (if divided into 8 bars)

Recipe 15: Cottage Cheese Pudding with Berries

Ingredients:
- Fat-free cottage cheese – 300 g (0.66 lb)
- Berries (raspberries, blueberries) – 150 g (0.33 lb)
- Honey – 30 g (0.07 lb)
- Vanilla extract – 1 teaspoon (about 5 ml or 0.17 oz)

Preparation Process:
1. In a bowl, mix cottage cheese, honey, and vanilla extract until smooth.
2. Divide the mixture into serving cups and top with berries.
3. Chill in the refrigerator for 1 hour before serving.

Yield:
- 450 g (0.99 lb)

Preparation Time:
- About 10 minutes + 1 hour chilling

Calories:
- Approximately 110 kcal per serving (if divided into 4 servings)

Recipe 16: Coconut Chocolate Cookies

Ingredients:
- Shredded coconut – 100 g (0.22 lb)
- Almond flour – 100 g (0.22 lb)
- Honey – 50 g (0.11 lb)
- Dark chocolate (70%) – 50 g (0.11 lb)

Preparation Process:
1. Preheat the oven to 180°C (350°F).
2. In a bowl, mix shredded coconut, almond flour, and honey to form a dough.
3. Shape into small balls and place on a baking sheet lined with parchment paper.
4. Bake for 12-15 minutes until golden brown.
5. Melt the chocolate in a double boiler and drizzle over the cookies.
6. Allow the chocolate to set before serving.

Yield:
- 250 g (0.55 lb)

Preparation Time:
- About 30 minutes

Calories:

- Approximately 100 kcal per cookie (if divided into 12 cookies)

Recipe 17: Kiwi Fruit Chips

Ingredients:

- Kiwis – 5 (about 500 g or 1.1 lb)
- Lemon juice – 1 tablespoon (about 15 ml or 0.5 oz)

Preparation Process:

1. Preheat the oven to 100°C (210°F).
2. Slice the kiwis thinly.
3. Place the slices on a baking sheet lined with parchment paper and drizzle with lemon juice.
4. Bake for 2-3 hours until fully dried.

Yield:

- 100 g (0.22 lb)

Preparation Time:

- About 3 hours

Calories:

- Approximately 50 kcal per 100 g

Recipe 18: Blueberry Crumble Pie

Ingredients:

- Blueberries – 400 g (0.88 lb)
- Oats – 150 g (0.33 lb)
- Whole wheat flour – 100 g (0.22 lb)
- Coconut oil – 50 g (0.11 lb)
- Honey – 50 g (0.11 lb)

Preparation Process:

1. Preheat the oven to 180°C (350°F).
2. In a bowl, mix oats, flour, coconut oil, and honey until crumbly.
3. Place blueberries in a baking dish and top with the oat crumble.
4. Bake for 25-30 minutes until golden brown.

Yield:

- 600 g (1.32 lb)

Preparation Time:

- About 40 minutes

Calories:

- Approximately 150 kcal per serving (if divided into 6 servings)

Recipe 19: Pear Salad with Nuts

Ingredients:

- Pears – 2 (about 300 g or 0.66 lb)
- Walnuts – 50 g (0.11 lb)
- Lettuce leaves – 100 g (0.22 lb)
- Lemon juice – 1 tablespoon (about 15 ml or 0.5 oz)
- Honey – 20 g (0.04 lb)

Preparation Process:

1. Slice the pears.
2. In a bowl, mix lemon juice and honey.
3. Arrange lettuce leaves on a plate, add pears and nuts.
4. Drizzle with the dressing and serve.

Yield:

- 450 g (0.99 lb)

Preparation Time:

- About 10 minutes

Calories:

- Approximately 120 kcal per serving (if divided into 4 servings)

Recipe 20: Baked Apples with Cinnamon and Honey

Ingredients:

- Apples – 4 (about 600 g or 1.32 lb)
- Cinnamon – 2 teaspoons (about 10 g or 0.02 lb)
- Honey – 40 g (0.09 lb)

Preparation Process:

1. Preheat the oven to 180°C (350°F).
2. Core the apples.
3. Place 1 teaspoon of honey and cinnamon inside each apple.
4. Place the apples on a baking sheet and bake for 25-30 minutes until tender.

Yield:

- 600 g (1.32 lb)

Preparation Time:

- About 35 minutes

Calories:

- Approximately 90 kcal per serving (if divided into 4 servings)

Recipe 21: Flourless Almond Cookies

Ingredients:

- Almond flour – 150 g (0.33 lb)
- Egg – 1
- Honey – 30 g (0.07 lb)
- Vanilla extract – 1 teaspoon (about 5 ml or 0.17 oz)

Preparation Process:

1. Preheat the oven to 180°C (350°F).
2. In a bowl, mix almond flour, egg, honey, and vanilla extract until well combined.
3. Shape into cookies and place on a baking sheet lined with parchment paper.
4. Bake for 10-12 minutes until golden brown.

Yield:

- 200 g (0.44 lb)

Preparation Time:

- About 20 minutes

Calories:

- Approximately 90 kcal per cookie (if divided into 10 cookies)

Recipe 22: Crustless Pumpkin Pie

Ingredients:

- Pumpkin puree – 400 g (0.88 lb)
- Eggs – 2
- Coconut milk – 200 ml (6.76 oz)
- Honey – 60 g (0.13 lb)
- Cinnamon – 1 teaspoon (about 5 g or 0.01 lb)

Preparation Process:

1. Preheat the oven to 180°C (350°F).
2. In a bowl, mix pumpkin puree, eggs, coconut milk, honey, and cinnamon.
3. Pour the mixture into a baking dish and bake for 45-50 minutes until fully set.

Yield:

- 600 g (1.32 lb)

Preparation Time:

- About 1 hour

- Approximately 150 kcal per serving (if divided into 6 servings)

Recipe 23: Oat Pancakes with Berries

Ingredients:

- Oats – 100 g (0.22 lb)
- Eggs – 2
- Almond milk – 100 ml (3.38 oz)
- Berries (of choice) – 100 g (0.22 lb)
- Honey – 30 g (0.07 lb)

Preparation Process:

1. Blend the oats into a flour-like consistency.
2. Mix oat flour, eggs, and almond milk in a bowl.
3. Cook pancakes on a lightly oiled pan.
4. Serve with berries and honey.

Yield:

- 400 g (0.88 lb)

Preparation Time:

- About 20 minutes

Calories:

- Approximately 120 kcal per serving (if divided into 4 servings)

Recipe 24: Granola with Honey and Nuts

Ingredients:

- Oats – 200 g (0.44 lb)
- Nuts (almonds, walnuts) – 100 g (0.22 lb)
- Honey – 50 g (0.11 lb)
- Coconut oil – 30 g (0.07 lb)
- Dried berries (cranberries, raisins) – 50 g (0.11 lb)

Preparation Process:

1. Preheat the oven to 150°C (300°F).
2. Mix oats and nuts in a bowl.
3. Melt honey and coconut oil in a saucepan, then combine with the oat mixture.
4. Spread the mixture on a baking sheet and bake for 20-25 minutes, stirring occasionally.
5. Add dried berries after baking.

Yield:
- 350 g (0.77 lb)

Preparation Time:
- About 30 minutes

Calories:
- Approximately 200 kcal per serving (if divided into 7 servings)

Recipe 25: Carrot Muffins

Ingredients:
- Grated carrot – 200 g (0.44 lb)
- Almond flour – 100 g (0.22 lb)
- Eggs – 2
- Honey – 50 g (0.11 lb)
- Baking powder – 1 teaspoon (about 5 g or 0.01 lb)

Preparation Process:
1. Preheat the oven to 180°C (350°F).
2. Mix all ingredients until well combined.
3. Divide the batter among muffin tins.
4. Bake for 20-25 minutes until golden brown.

Yield:
- 300 g (0.66 lb)

Preparation Time:
- About 30 minutes

Calories:
- Approximately 100 kcal per muffin (if divided into 8 muffins)

Recipe 26: Strawberry Parfait with Yogurt

Ingredients:
- Strawberries – 200 g (0.44 lb)
- Natural yogurt – 200 g (0.44 lb)
- Honey – 30 g (0.07 lb)
- Granola – 50 g (0.11 lb)

Preparation Process:
1. Slice the strawberries.
2. Layer yogurt, strawberries, honey, and granola in glasses.
3. Chill in the refrigerator before serving.

Yield:

- 400 g (0.88 lb)

Preparation Time:

- About 10 minutes

Calories:

- Approximately 150 kcal per serving (if divided into 4 servings)

Recipe 27: No-Bake Lemon Cheesecake

Ingredients:

- Cream cheese – 200 g (0.44 lb)
- Greek yogurt – 150 g (0.33 lb)
- Honey – 50 g (0.11 lb)
- Lemon juice – 2 tablespoons (about 30 ml or 1 oz)
- Gelatin – 10 g (0.02 lb)

Preparation Process:

1. Mix cream cheese, yogurt, honey, and lemon juice until smooth.
2. Dissolve gelatin in a small amount of hot water and add to the mixture.
3. Pour the mixture into a mold and chill in the refrigerator until set (about 2 hours).

Yield:

- 400 g (0.88 lb)

Preparation Time:

- About 15 minutes + chilling time

Calories:

- Approximately 180 kcal per serving (if divided into 4 servings)

Recipe 28: Orange Mousse

Ingredients:

- Oranges – 4 (about 600 g or 1.32 lb)
- Greek yogurt – 200 g (0.44 lb)
- Honey – 50 g (0.11 lb)
- Gelatin – 10 g (0.02 lb)

Preparation Process:

1. Squeeze the juice from the oranges.
2. Mix yogurt, honey, and orange juice in a bowl.

3. Dissolve gelatin in a small amount of hot water and add to the mixture.
4. Pour the mousse into serving glasses and refrigerate until set (about 2 hours).

Yield:
- 500 g (1.1 lb)

Preparation Time:
- About 15 minutes + chilling time

Calories:
- Approximately 140 kcal per serving (if divided into 4 servings)

Recipe 29: Blueberry-Almond Energy Balls

Ingredients:
- Ground almonds – 100 g (0.22 lb)
- Blueberries (fresh or dried) – 100 g (0.22 lb)
- Oats – 50 g (0.11 lb)
- Honey – 30 g (0.07 lb)
- Coconut oil – 20 g (0.04 lb)
- Vanilla extract – 1 teaspoon (about 5 ml or 0.17 oz)

Preparation Process:
1. Blend the oats and almonds into a flour-like consistency.
2. Add blueberries, honey, coconut oil, and vanilla extract. Blend until well combined.
3. Form the mixture into small balls.
4. Refrigerate the balls for 1-2 hours to set.

Yield:
- 250 g (0.55 lb)

Preparation Time:
- About 15 minutes + chilling time

Calories:
- Approximately 50 kcal per ball (if divided into 10 balls)

Recipe 30: Coconut Mango Treats

Ingredients:
- Shredded coconut – 150 g (0.33 lb)
- Fresh mango – 200 g (0.44 lb)
- Coconut milk – 100 ml (3.38 oz)
- Honey – 40 g (0.09 lb)

- Oat flour – 50 g (0.11 lb)

Preparation Process:

1. Dice the mango into small cubes.
2. Mix shredded coconut, oat flour, and honey in a bowl.
3. Add coconut milk and mango, and mix until you have a uniform dough.
4. Press the dough into a mold and smooth it out.
5. Chill in the refrigerator for at least 2 hours.
6. Cut into small portions before serving.

Yield:

- 400 g (0.88 lb)

Preparation Time:

- About 20 minutes + chilling time

Calories:

- Approximately 180 kcal per serving (if divided into 4 servings)

Conclusion

Healthy eating is not just a set of rules or restrictions; it's a lifestyle that brings joy, energy, and long-term well-being. Through this journey, you've discovered not only new flavors and recipes but also the importance of taking care of your body through nutrition. Each step you've taken brings you closer to a healthier, happier, and more active life.

Remember, perfection is not about completely changing your diet in one day but about making small, mindful steps towards your goals. Don't be afraid to experiment, listen to your body, and find pleasure in each meal. Health is about balance, and it's up to you to create a diet that supports you both physically and emotionally.

With this book, you've not only learned how to eat properly but also gained a powerful tool for creating a new, improved version of yourself.

May your journey to health and fitness be smooth, delicious, and full of inspiration.

Live enjoying your food and taking care of your body, as health is the most valuable gift you can give yourself.

On this path, you are not alone, and we are delighted to be your companion on the road to a healthy and fulfilling lifestyle!